How I Overcame Hypothyroidism

How I Overcame Hypothyroidism

Dr. Ray Peat's Principles for Metabolic and Hormonal Regeneration

Benedicte Mai Lerche MSc PhD

BiochemNordic

"Healing Metabolism"

Book 1

A note to the reader:
The author of this book shares their personal experience in utilizing Dr. Ray Peat's health principles, which are considered controversial, with differing opinions among experts. The information provided is not intended to diagnose, treat, cure, or prevent any diseases or health problems. Neither the author nor the publisher makes any express or implied representations or warranties regarding the information's suitability, reliability, timeliness, or accuracy. The author and publisher assume no responsibility for any consequences resulting from the readers' use or misuse of the information presented. Specifically, they disclaim any responsibility for personal or other liability, loss, or risk that may be incurred as a consequence, directly or indirectly, of using or applying any of the contents of this book. The information shared should not be regarded as a substitute for professional medical advice or treatment. It is strongly recommended that readers seek the guidance of a qualified healthcare provider for any questions or concerns regarding their health or medical condition. Readers should be aware that the decision to incorporate this information into their own lives is their own choice and responsibility. They bear sole responsibility for adhering to the laws of their respective state and country regarding the purchase and consumption of any food, medication, hormone, or supplement.

Book Series

Through my "Healing Metabolism" book series, I am dedicated to sharing Dr. Ray Peat's health research. The series aims to deepen readers' understanding and offer practical methods for overcoming metabolic and hormonal imbalances, utilizing diet, thyroid replacement therapy, hormonal support compounds, and other lifestyle changes.

Book 1:

The current book, "How I Overcame Hypothyroidism," chronicles my personal health journey and victory over low thyroid function (hypothyroidism) using Dr. Ray Peat's health approach. It introduces Dr. Peat's research and equips readers with a fundamental understanding of his key health concepts for healing metabolism.

Book 2:

The second book, "Test Your Thyroid Function," delves into Dr. Ray Peat's principles for thyroid testing and the diagnosis of hypothyroidism. This volume provides crucial knowledge for understanding thyroid blood tests and explains how to use pulse rate and body temperature to track your metabolism at home. Additionally, it covers essential aspects of thyroid function and metabolic health.

Book 3:

The third book "How To Boost Metabolism With Food" explores Dr. Ray Peat's nutritional research, offering a detailed and approachable explanation of his pro-metabolic diet principles.

Future volumes:

I am developing further volumes for the "Healing Metabolism" series. Upcoming books will provide insights into topics such as thyroid medication and hormonal support supplements like progesterone and pregnenolone.

Support my work:

If you find any of my books helpful, I would be extremely grateful if you could take a few minutes to leave a short review on the platform where you purchased the book or on Goodreads. This will help other potential readers dealing with similar health issues discover and benefit from my work.

Contents

Dedication

With deep appreciation, this book is dedicated to the late Dr. Ray Peat, whose exceptional research and generous support profoundly transformed my life and restored my health.

Raymond Franklin Peat (1936-2022), a distinguished American researcher with a Ph.D. in biology, devoted over five decades to the study of nutrition and hormones. His pioneering work on diet, metabolism, progesterone, and related hormones has left an indelible impact on these fields.

Dr. Ray Peat's unwavering commitment to balancing thyroid function resonated deeply with me, and his groundbreaking research has positively influenced the lives of numerous individuals, including myself.

Within the pages of this book, I recount my journey, navigating the challenges of addressing my low thyroid symptoms and Dr. Ray Peat's pivotal role in redirecting my path, ultimately saving my health.

Through this book, I aim to provide an accessible introduction to Dr. Ray Peat's invaluable health principles, encompassing the practical steps he imparted to me for achieving harmony in thyroid function and hormones.

Benedicte Mai Lerche
August 2023

Introduction

Throughout my early twenties, I faced the daunting challenge of severe hypothyroidism, grappling with debilitating symptoms and struggling to find effective treatment. It was during this difficult period that I embarked on a personal journey that would ultimately change the course of my life.

In my quest for answers and relief, I discovered the groundbreaking research of Dr. Ray Peat, a renowned expert in the field of nutrition, metabolism, and hormones.

Dr. Peat's health principles and insights became the turning point in my battle against hypothyroidism, empowering me to regain control of my health and well-being.

Inspired by my own transformation, I decided to study biochemistry at university and eventually created my website, biochemnordic.com. Through this platform, I began sharing my experiences using Dr. Ray Peat's health principles and providing nutritional and metabolic counseling to others struggling with thyroid and hormonal issues.

As I connected with more individuals, I realized that my story was not unique. Many others were grappling with similar health challenges, desperately seeking solutions to alleviate their low thyroid symptoms. This realization has kept compelling me to take action and develop and improve the information I share through my website.

My book series 'Healing Metabolism' serves as another way of bridging the gap between those suffering from hypothyroidism and the transformative knowledge of Dr. Ray Peat.

My goal with this first volume is to provide a comprehensive and accessible introduction to his research, thereby equipping individuals with the information they need to heal and restore balance to their thyroid function and hormones.

The book presents a detailed account of my own experience, revealing the challenges I faced within the realm of conventional medicine and the arduous process of trial and error that ultimately led me to Dr. Ray Peat's invaluable work.
I will provide insights into my personal application of Dr. Ray Peat's teachings, and explain the exact steps I took to overcome hypothyroidism.

It is my sincere hope that this book serves as a guiding light for those navigating the complex world of hypothyroidism, enabling them to embark on their own path toward metabolic and hormonal regeneration.

The book is organized as follows:

Chapter 1: In this chapter, I recount my personal experience of falling ill, navigating the conventional medical system, and receiving a diagnosis of hypothyroidism. I also discuss the various treatments I tried before discovering Dr. Ray Peat's research.

Chapter 2: This chapter explores different aspects of thyroid function and metabolism, highlighting the significant consequences of hypothyroidism, including its common symptoms and triggers.

Chapter 3: Here, I delve into Dr. Ray Peat's perspective on thyroid testing, explaining his expert guidance on thyroid blood tests and his emphasis on using pulse rate and body temperature as indicators of thyroid function.

Chapter 4: This chapter focuses on Dr. Peat's dietary recommendations. I discuss the fundamental principles of his pro-metabolic diet, including his suggestions for fats, proteins, and carbohydrates. I explain the detrimental effects of an improper diet on thyroid function. Additionally, I outline the benefits of Dr. Peat's renowned carrot salad and the importance of stabilizing blood sugar levels and creating well-balanced meals.

Chapter 5: In this chapter, I explore Dr. Ray Peat's suggestions for thyroid medication. I address the limitations of the common T4 treatment approach and explain how Dr. Ray Peat guided me in incorporating a combination of both T4 and T3 in my treatment regimen.

Chapter 6: This chapter delves into Dr. Ray Peat's insights on protective natural hormones like progesterone and pregnenolone. I discuss the anti-aging and anti-stress properties of these hormones and explain how I integrated them into my recovery process.

Chapter 7: Here, the focus is on nutritional supplements. I discuss Dr. Ray Peat's perspective on the potential dangers of fillers and binders in supplements, as well as the associated risks of certain nutritional supplements. I share my personal experience of modifying my supplement regimen based on Dr. Ray's recommendations.

Chapter 8: In this chapter, the focus is on the importance of light therapy. I explain how prolonged periods of darkness can negatively impact health. Furthermore, I explore the potential benefits of sunlight exposure and discuss how the use of red and orange light therapy lamps can contribute to improved hormonal balance.

Chapter 9: Finally, in this chapter, I recount my journey toward achieving complete recovery and my ongoing commitment to staying informed about Dr. Ray Peat's research. I delve into the successful integration of his health principles into my life over the years.

Benedicte Mai Lerche MSc PhD

Chapter 1: My Health Story

How I Became Ill

After completing high school in my home country, Denmark, I had the opportunity to work as an au pair for a French family in Paris. My primary duties involved taking care of their two children and handling various household chores. Additionally, I attended a language school to improve my French language skills.

The family I worked for generously provided a separate apartment for the au pair, which was wonderful as it granted me privacy during weekends. However, the apartment was situated in an old building that was riddled with mold. This environment had a detrimental impact on my health, and within a few months of staying there, I began experiencing a range of health issues.

I developed symptoms such as frequent colds, respiratory infections, digestive problems including constipation, and intense pain and bloating after meals. Moreover, I suffered from debilitating fatigue, muscle pain, headaches, dizziness, nasal congestion, dry skin, skin rashes, and thinning hair. Additionally, my menstrual cycles become irregular, and I experienced a prolonged absence of my period.

My Medical Journey

I sought medical assistance in France to address my deteriorating health issues. However, despite undergoing various tests, the doctors were unable to identify the underlying cause of my wide range of symptoms. As a remedy, they prescribed a birth control pill to regulate my menstrual cycle and provided recommendations for managing my digestive problems.

Unfortunately, my symptoms continued to worsen, forcing me to return home to Denmark a few months earlier than planned. I had hoped that being back home and away from the moldy apartment would facilitate my recovery. However, even after several months back in Denmark, my symptoms persisted.

In light of this, I sought medical advice from doctors in Denmark and underwent additional tests. These tests revealed that I had high blood cholesterol, polycystic ovarian syndrome (PCOS), and severe hypoglycemia (low blood sugar). Later, I discovered from Dr. Ray Peat that these health issues are associated with an underactive thyroid function.

Surprisingly, most of my blood tests for thyroid function fell within the normal range. It is a common occurrence for individuals to experience low thyroid symptoms despite having normal thyroid function test results. I will delve further into this topic later in this book.

Despite undergoing numerous tests, the doctors were unable to identify the underlying cause or provide a diagnosis for my multiple persistent symptoms. This frustrating process lasted over a year, hindering my ability to begin university studies. Even when I attempted to commence my studies, the severity of headaches, fatigue, dizziness, low blood sugar, digestive pain, and muscle pain made concentration impossible, leading me to discontinue my education.

Silent Struggles

As a young individual with undiagnosed hypothyroidism, I faced various challenges. I was unable to pursue a university education like my peers, and I encountered difficulties in engaging in typical social activities. Frequently, I had to decline invitations from friends and family due to my compromised health.

Unfortunately, in my experience, many individuals with undiagnosed hypothyroidism suffer from severe symptoms that hinder their ability to work, study, or engage in social interactions.

Motivated by the desperate need for symptom relief and growing frustration with conventional medical treatments, I invested a significant amount of money in alternative therapies. These included approaches such as homeopathy, high-dose vitamin and mineral regimens, and specialized diets targeting issues like candida overgrowth and parasites. Regrettably, none of these methods yielded positive results.

Through my work as a nutritional and metabolic counselor, I have personally witnessed the silent suffering of numerous individuals living with undiagnosed hypothyroidism. It is truly heart-wrenching to witness people losing hope and depleting their hard-earned funds on ineffective treatments. Consequently, they are left feeling defeated, which creates substantial barriers to trust in new and potentially beneficial approaches.

This is precisely why I wrote this book - to serve as a beacon of hope for those grappling with low thyroid function. The book encompasses a holistic yet scientific approach to overcoming hypothyroidism and restoring hormonal balance.

My Thyroid Diagnosis

When I was exploring alternative treatments to alleviate my symptoms, I experienced increasing frustration. Many of the treatments I encountered seemed unscientific and lacked credibility, leaving me with a sense of hopelessness and confusion.

However, by a stroke of luck, I crossed paths with an individual who had a background in dentistry and extensive knowledge about vitamins and minerals. After assessing my symptoms, he suggested that I might be dealing with underactive thyroid function, which sparked a glimmer of hope that I could finally find some relief.

Following his advice, I sought out a specialized medical clinic in Denmark. There, I underwent additional thyroid tests and completed a comprehensive questionnaire about my symptoms. It was during this process that I received the diagnosis of hypothyroidism, and for the first time, I felt like I had some clarity regarding my long-standing health issues. Initially, I was grateful for the diagnosis and optimistic that the clinic would provide effective treatment for my condition.

However, my hopes were soon shattered as I discovered that the clinic lacked the necessary expertise to effectively address my condition. They prescribed thyroid medication, but unfortunately, it only exacerbated my symptoms, leaving me feeling exhausted and experiencing severe headaches and water retention.

Through my personal experiences and counseling others, I have learned that initiating thyroid medication can be a challenging process for individuals with severe hypothyroidism. Gradually increasing the dosage is crucial to avoid adverse reactions, a topic that I will delve into further in this book.

Feeling dissatisfied with the medical clinic's ability to assist me, I turned to the internet in search of more information on treating underactive thyroid function.

It was during this exploration that I came across Dr. Ray Peat's work. This discovery became a turning point in my healing journey, providing me with the strength and determination to take charge of my health and find the much-needed relief I had been desperately seeking.

Finding Dr. Ray Peat

Upon discovering the groundbreaking research of Dr. Ray Peat, it became evident to me that his information was unparalleled among other resources found on the internet and surpassed the level of comprehensiveness provided by the medical clinic that initially diagnosed me with low thyroid function.

Motivated by this realization, I reached out to Dr. Peat, who graciously assisted me in gaining a deeper understanding of my body's inner workings and how hypothyroidism served as the root cause of my symptoms.

I discovered that the moldy and dark apartment in Paris, coupled with the recurring colds and respiratory infections, had contributed to the decline in my thyroid function. Dr. Ray Peat explained how hypothyroidism was responsible for my elevated cholesterol levels, hypoglycemia, polycystic ovaries (PCO), fatigue, headaches, digestive issues, and muscle pain.

To gain a deeper understanding of Dr. Ray Peat's approach, I acquired and read all of his books and subscribed to his newsletter. Armed with this wealth of material and Dr. Ray Peat's compassionate support and guidance on diet, thyroid medication, nutritional supplements, and hormonal support compounds my health improved remarkably.

Within a few months, I regained sufficient well-being to commence my studies in biochemistry at the University of Copenhagen.

Over the years, I maintained regular contact with Dr. Ray Peat and closely followed his ongoing research. Consistently applying his health principles has resulted in astounding success, leaving me truly amazed. The continued efficacy of his principles never ceases to astound me.

As a biochemist, I have developed a profound appreciation for the exceptional fusion of scientific and holistic approaches in Dr. Ray Peat's health paradigm.

Unlike conventional medicine, which often views the body as a collection of disconnected parts, Dr. Ray Peat's research interconnects these facets in a comprehensive and scientific manner, providing a deeper understanding of the root cause behind symptoms.

Rather than merely addressing isolated symptoms, Dr. Ray Peat's approach concentrates on rectifying the underlying imbalances.

It is crucial to understand that Dr. Ray Peat's health principles do not offer a quick fix but rather represent a long-term lifestyle choice grounded in a profound comprehension of the body's biochemical workings.

If you choose to embrace his health methodology for healing your thyroid and restoring hormonal balance, it requires a commitment to sustained implementation.

In the upcoming pages, I will introduce you to Dr. Ray Peat's teachings. We will delve into different aspects of thyroid function and metabolism, uncovering the significant consequences of hypothyroidism. Alongside that, I will share my personal experience of utilizing Dr. Peat's teachings to address my own challenges with low thyroid function and hormonal imbalances.

Together, we will explore Dr. Peat's guidance on thyroid function assessment, dietary recommendations, thyroid medication, nutritional supplements, hormonal support, and light therapy.

Through this exploration, you will gain valuable insights into Dr. Peat's principles for metabolic and hormonal regeneration.

Chapter 2: Thyroid Function

The Thyroid Gland

Thyroid function refers to metabolism or the metabolic rate, which is a medical term indicating the process through which cells convert food (nutrients) into energy (Barnes & Galton, 1976, p. 3).

Thyroid function is regulated by the thyroid hormones, which are produced and released by the thyroid gland (Society of Endocrinology, 2020).

Located in the front of the throat, the human thyroid gland has a butterfly shape (Barnes & Galton, 1976, p. 3). It is a small endocrine gland that produces and releases triiodothyronine (T3), the active thyroid hormone, and thyroxine (T4), a prohormone or storage hormone. Collectively, T4 and T3 are known as the thyroid hormones (Society of Endocrinology, 2020).

Once secreted by the thyroid gland, T4 can be converted to the active thyroid hormone T3 by specific enzymes in other organs and tissues (Society of Endocrinology, 2020). Most of this conversion occurs in the liver, which allows the liver to regulate thyroid function (Peat, 2001a, p. 73).

There is an interrelationship between the thyroid gland and other endocrine glands. The function of the thyroid gland affects the adrenals, pancreas, and sex glands, meaning the ovaries and testes (Barnes & Galton, 1976, p. 20).

It is important to note that there is a lack of clarity in the literature regarding the ratio of T4 to T3 secreted by the human thyroid gland.

Some studies indicate that the gland secretes about 80% T4 and 20% T3, resulting in a T4 to T3 ratio of 4:1 (Society of Endocrinology, 2020).

However, other researchers argue that the gland primarily secretes T4 and only a small amount of T3, suggesting a ratio of 13 to 1 of T4 to T3 (Wiersinga et al., 2012, p. 62).

As per Dr. Ray Peat, the human thyroid gland releases T4 and T3 in a ratio of 3:1, which corresponds to 75% T4 and 25% T3 (Peat, 2001a, p. 73). Consequently, in this book, I will adopt the premise that the human thyroid gland secretes T4 and T3 in a 3:1 ratio.

Understanding the ratio of T4 to T3 secreted by the human thyroid gland is essential as it serves as the foundation for determining the appropriate thyroid replacement therapy using these hormones (Peat, 2000, p. 5). I will revisit this topic later in this book.

The Active Thyroid Hormone

When discussing thyroid function, it is essential to keep in mind that T3 serves as the active thyroid hormone, while T4 is a storage hormone that acts as a prohormone for T3 (Society of Endocrinology, 2020).

The primary role of T3 is to provide energy to cells, enabling the body's tissues and organs to carry out vital life processes (Vander et al., 2001, p. 267).

T3 exerts a significant influence on nearly all physiological processes within the body, including metabolism, growth and development, body temperature, and heart rate. T3 also plays a crucial role in cellular differentiation, enabling cells to carry out specialized functions (Vander et al., 2001, pp. 619-620). Additionally, T3 contributes to the maintenance of a healthy circulatory system, appropriate blood volume, and optimal nerve and muscle function (Barnes & Galton, 1976, p. 3).

One specific aspect controlled by T3 is the metabolic rate, which refers to the speed at which cells utilize oxygen to convert nutrients into carbon dioxide, water, heat, and ATP (adenosine triphosphate) - a biological form of energy (Vander et al., 2001, pp. 619-620).

ATP acts as an energy source within the body, powering essential cellular functions and reactions (Vander et al., 2001, pp. 619-620).

Peat emphasized the necessity of abundant energy for maintaining the proper structure and function of the body's tissues and organs (Peat, 2001a, pp. 1-5). He argued that since T3 controls the body's energy production, improving thyroid function has the potential to address a range of health problems (Peat, 2001a, pp. 1-5).

This understanding held immense importance for me, as I finally comprehended how hypothyroidism contributes to a multitude of issues. It became clear that restoring my thyroid function was essential for recovering my overall health.

What is Hypothyroidism?

Hypothyroidism, also known as low thyroid function, can occur due to various factors. These factors include inadequate production of thyroid hormones by the thyroid gland, ineffective conversion of T4 to T3 in the organs and tissues, or impaired cellular response to T3 (Peat, 2001a, pp. 72-74; Wilson, 2015, pp. 24-28). Dr. Ray Peat's extensive research suggests that hypothyroidism usually arises from a combination of these factors. Regardless of the underlying cause, hypothyroidism ultimately leads to a deficiency of energy (Peat, 2001a, pp. 72-74; Peat, 2008, pp. 2-3).

Peat suggested that it is an imbalance between the body's energy resources and the demands imposed on it by the environment that creates diseases (Peat, 2001a, pp. 1-5). He explained that hypothyroidism, characterized by low energy levels, plays a significant role in initiating detrimental degenerative processes. Since hypothyroidism affects all cells and tissues in the body, it manifests in various symptoms (Peat, 2001d, p. 16).

The severe forms of hypothyroidism, known as cretinism in infants and children, and myxedema in adults, are recognized for their profound impact on the body, affecting all tissues and organs and leading to devastating outcomes (Barnes & Galton, 1976, pp. 20-22). However, it is important to note that severe hypothyroidism is relatively uncommon (Barnes & Galton, 1976, pp. 20-22).

On the other hand, milder forms of hypothyroidism are prevalent but can present with subtle symptoms. It may affect various body systems, though not necessarily to the same degree in each individual. Manifestations of hypothyroidism can differ from person to person (Barnes & Galton, 1976, pp. 22-25).

In fact, it is not uncommon to have hypothyroidism without being aware of it. This lack of awareness may have led to attempts to manage individual symptoms without identifying the underlying cause.

Symptoms of Hypothyroidism

Below is a list of common symptoms associated with hypothyroidism (Barnes & Galton, 1976, pp. 22-24; Wilson, 2015, p. 25; Peat, 2001d, pp. 16-18; Peat, 2001b, p. 78).

While not exhaustive, the list provides an overview of the diverse symptoms related to low thyroid function. It is important to note that not all symptoms need to be present for a diagnosis of hypothyroidism

List of symptoms associated with hypothyroidism:

Fatigue: Feeling tired and lacking energy, even after getting adequate rest (chronic fatigue).

Headaches: Experiencing pressure headaches and migraines.

Hypoglycemia: Having low blood sugar, resulting in a need to eat frequently to avoid feeling faint and dizzy.

Weight changes: Experiencing unexplained weight gain or difficulty losing weight despite maintaining a healthy diet and regular exercise routine. Some individuals may also experience weight loss.

Low body temperature: Having cold intolerance, feeling excessively cold even in warm temperatures, and having cold hands and feet.

Reduced heart rate: Experiencing a slow heart rate (bradycardia) and decreased heart function.

Heart problems & disease: Experiencing heart pain, poor heart sounds, enlargement of the heart, palpitations, and hypertension.

Constipation: Experiencing slow digestion, difficulty passing stools, and infrequent bowel movements.

Digestive problems: Painful digestion, irritable bowel syndrome (IBS), as well as an overgrowth of bad bacteria and candida.

Dry skin: Having dry, rough, thin, pale skin that may be itchy and scaly, accompanied by conditions like eczema or skin infections.

Brittle hair & nails: Experiencing thinning of hair and nails, hair loss, changes in hair texture, and potential loss of the outer third of the eyebrows.

Muscle and joint pain: Experiencing muscle aches, stiffness, and joint pain not attributed to any specific injury or physical activity.

Carpal tunnel syndrome: Having pain, numbness, and tingling sensations in the hand, arms, and fingers (carpal tunnel syndrome).

Mood changes: Experiencing depression, anxiety, irritability, and mood swings.

Cognitive impairment: Having difficulty concentrating, poor memory, and decreased mental alertness (brain fog).

Hoarseness: Experiencing a deepening or hoarse voice, often accompanied by a sore throat.

Swelling: Experiencing water retention (edema), often with swelling or puffiness in the face, hands, feet, or ankles.

High cholesterol: Having elevated levels of cholesterol in the blood, even with a healthy diet and lifestyle.

Decreased libido: Experiencing a loss of interest in sexual activity and a reduced sexual drive.

Menstrual irregularities: Having irregular menstrual cycles, heavy menstrual bleeding, prolonged menstrual periods, painful menstruation, and experiencing symptoms of premenstrual syndrome (PMS) and polycystic ovaries (PCOS).

Infertility & miscarriage: Experiencing male and female infertility, with a higher chance of miscarriage in females.

Insomnia: Having problems falling asleep and/or waking up during the night.

Other symptoms: Poor vision, hearing loss, anemia, allergies, frequent colds, infections, orange calluses, inflammation, premature aging, and more.

Triggers of Hypothyroidism

Based on my experience working with clients, I have noticed that an improper diet and various forms of mental or physical stress are commonly implicated as triggers for developing hypothyroidism.

Fasting, chronic protein deficiency, consumption of foods known to be detrimental to the thyroid, as well as stress arising from excessive aerobic exercise, work overload, challenging relationships, or severe bacterial or viral infections, are often recurring factors among individuals who develop hypothyroidism.

Many health-conscious individuals may unknowingly adopt a diet and lifestyle that worsen hypothyroidism. This can include engaging in intense exercise that leaves one breathless and consuming foods such as beans, lentils, nuts, polyunsaturated fats, and undercooked broccoli, cauliflower, cabbage, or mustard greens, all of which inhibit thyroid function (Peat, 2001a, p. 75).

Although individuals may have mildly low thyroid levels in their medical history, significant issues may not arise until they adopt an improper diet or encounter stressors.

From my personal perspective, I suspect that I have been dealing with hypothyroidism since birth, considering my history of food allergies and severe eczema during childhood, as well as the symptoms of fatigue, weight gain, constipation, and ongoing food allergies I experienced throughout my teenage years.

I believe that my hypothyroidism developed due to my poor dietary choices, as well as the stressors of living in a dark and moldy apartment and experiencing recurrent flu-like infections.

It is plausible that you, too, are following an improper diet and have experienced stress that has triggered your thyroid issues.

Dr. Ray Peat explained the importance of not fixating excessively on the specific triggers that caused hypothyroidism. It's common for individuals, including myself, to give excessive attention to factors like mold exposure or viral and bacterial infections. However, it is crucial to shift the focus away from continuously trying to treat these specific issues. Instead, the key lies in removing oneself from an unfavorable environment and dedicating efforts towards practices that improve thyroid function and hormonal balance. By adopting this approach, individuals can optimize their body's healing capabilities.

For a deeper understanding of crucial elements related to hypothyroidism and overall thyroid well-being, I recommend consulting my book, "Test Your Thyroid Function."

Chapter 3: Thyroid Testing

Thyroid Blood Tests

Blood tests play a crucial role in assessing thyroid function, but it is essential to consider various factors before solely relying on the results.

Firstly, it is important to understand the issues surrounding the reference ranges for thyroid blood tests (Peat, 2008, p. 2). Additionally, blood tests may not accurately reflect cellular thyroid function as they measure hormone levels in the blood rather than how these hormones affect the cells (Peat, 2001a, p. 72; Wilson, 2015, p. 28).

When evaluating thyroid function, doctors typically conduct blood tests for TSH, T4, and T3 hormones (Peat, 2008, p. 2; Peat, 2001a, p. 74).

Dr. Ray Peat emphasized that the reference ranges for T4 and T3 have been standardized based on individuals taking a thyroxine (T4) medication (Peat, 2000, p. 5). However, it is important to know that healthy individuals who do not take any thyroid medication typically have a higher ratio of T3 to T4 compared to those taking thyroxine (Peat, 2000, p. 5; Wiersinga et al., 2012, p. 62).

Thyroid-stimulating hormone (TSH), released by the pituitary gland in the brain, stimulates the thyroid gland to produce and release thyroid hormones

(Vander et al., 2001, p. 280; Society of Endocrinology, 2020).

The thyroid hormones and TSH have a negative feedback relationship. If the TSH value is low, it indicates that the blood levels of T4 and T3 are adequate. Conversely, when the levels of T4 and T3 are low, the TSH increases (Vander et al., 2001, p. 281). Consequently, the TSH value is utilized as a means to evaluate the function of the thyroid gland (Vander et al., 2001, p. 281; Peat, 2008, p. 2).
The crucial point is then to determine the threshold level of TSH that indicates the presence of hypothyroidism (Peat, 2008, p. 2). However, experts disagree about the appropriate upper limit for TSH (Faix, 2013).

In many countries, the upper limit for TSH is approximately 4 mIU/L (Faix, 2013). In 2003, the American Association of Clinical Endocrinologists updated its guidelines for the reference range of TSH to 0.3-3 mIU/L (Peat, 2008, p. 2). Some experts suggest that the upper limit for TSH should be set even lower, around 2.5 mIU/L (Faix, 2013). Dr. Ray Peat advocated for a TSH level below 1 mIU/L (Peat, 2008, p. 2). He emphasized that many symptoms of hypothyroidism are actually connected to the elevated TSH itself (Peat, 2008, p. 2).

Further complicating the situation is the fact that high levels of the stress hormone cortisol can inhibit the secretion of thyroid-stimulating hormone (TSH), creating a scenario where TSH levels may appear normal or even low despite the presence of actual hypothyroidism (Peat, 2008, p. 3). Therefore, relying solely on TSH as an indicator of thyroid function can be misleading (Peat, 2008, p. 3).

In certain cases, individuals may exhibit above-average levels of T4 but still experience symptoms of hypothyroidism, which is likely due to an ineffective conversion of T4 to T3 (Peat, 2001a, p. 74). Women, in particular, may face challenges in converting T4 to the active thyroid hormone T3 due to lower liver activity influenced, in part, by excess estrogen that inhibits liver function (Peat, 2001a, p. 74).

Stress not only suppresses TSH but also exerts additional effects in inhibiting proper thyroid function. Cortisol and adrenaline, which are both stress hormones, inhibit the conversion of T4 to T3 (Peat, 2008, p. 3). Additionally, adrenaline increases the production of reverse T3 (rT3), an inactive form of T3 that interferes with the functionality of T3 (Peat, 2008, p. 3; Peat, 2001d, p. 20).

Various other factors, such as low blood sugar, insufficient dietary protein, or certain mineral deficiencies, can also contribute to the inadequate conversion of T4 to T3 (Peat, 2001a, pp. 73-75; Wilson, 2015, p. 26). Furthermore, the response of tissues to the active T3 hormone can be suppressed, for example, by polyunsaturated fats (Peat, 2001a, p. 72).

Peat's work emphasizes that true thyroid function at the cellular level is significantly influenced by various factors, including stress, estrogen, diet, digestion, and more. This complexity makes it challenging to accurately predict actual thyroid function based solely on blood tests (Peat, 2001a, p. 72).

Consequently, in evaluating thyroid function, Dr. Ray Peat employed a comprehensive approach by combining blood test results with pulse and temperature measurements, as well as an assessment of a person's symptoms (Peat, 2008, p. 5). This same comprehensive approach is also applied when I help individuals evaluate their thyroid function.

Despite the numerous challenges associated with interpreting blood tests for thyroid function, it is crucial to consult with a doctor and undergo such tests if you suspect that you have a thyroid issue.

Thyroid blood tests are especially important before initiating any form of thyroid replacement therapy.

For individuals already undergoing thyroid replacement therapy, blood tests, along with the monitoring of symptoms, pulse rate, and body temperature, play a vital role in assessing the effectiveness of the treatment (Peat, 2008, p. 5).

For further understanding of thyroid blood tests, consider my book "Test Your Thyroid Function." This resource offers extensive knowledge, enabling you to effectively interpret your own thyroid blood test results.

Pulse and Temperature

Low body temperature is recognized as a significant indicator of hypothyroidism (Wilson, 2015, pp. 24-28; Barnes & Galton, 1976, p. 285).

Dr. Ray Peat employed both body temperature and pulse rate in the evaluation of thyroid function (Peat, 2001a, p. 72). According to Dr. Peat, these measurements offer valuable insights into thyroid function at the cellular level.

According to Peat (2008, p. 4), the combination of body temperature and pulse rate offers a more comprehensive assessment of thyroid function compared to either measurement alone.

Optimal thyroid function, as described by Peat, is characterized by an oral temperature of approximately 98.6°F (37°C) and a pulse rate ranging from 80 to 85 beats per minute (Peat, 2001b, p. 76). Upon waking, individuals with good thyroid function may experience slightly lower temperature and pulse, but these values should rise to the optimal range during mid-morning and remain elevated throughout the day (Peat, 2001b, p. 76).

In contrast, individuals with hypothyroidism often exhibit oral temperatures significantly below 98°F

(36.6°C) and pulse rates in the 60s or sometimes even 50s (Peat, 2001d, p. 17).

While a low pulse rate is typically associated with good health, it can also indicate low thyroid function (Peat, 2001d, p. 17). When low body temperature and pulse rate coincide with several symptoms of hypothyroidism, it strongly suggests the presence of a thyroid issue (Peat, 2001b, p. 76).

It is important to recognize that individuals with low thyroid function may compensate for the lack of energy by producing high levels of the stress hormones cortisol and adrenaline (Peat, 2008, p. 5).

The stress hormones can keep the temperature and pulse rate elevated, despite the presence of hypothyroidism, which can complicate the accurate measurement of thyroid function using pulse and temperature readings (Peat, 2008, p. 5).

According to Dr. Peat's findings (Peat, 2001a, p. 72; Peat, 2008, p. 5), individuals with hypothyroidism may exhibit adrenaline levels as much as 40 times higher than average. Consequently, this leads to a notable increase in pulse rate.

After eating breakfast, stress hormones begin to return to normal. Consequently, taking pulse and temperature measurements before and after breakfast can help differentiate between stress levels and actual thyroid function (Peat, 2008, p. 5).

I have incorporated Dr. Ray Peat's pulse and temperature method, alongside symptom assessment and thyroid blood tests, to evaluate my own thyroid function and gauge the effectiveness of my thyroid replacement therapy throughout the years. When providing guidance to individuals, I strongly encourage them to follow a similar approach, as it can provide valuable insights into their thyroid function.

If you're looking to gain further understanding and guidance of how to assess your thyroid function using body temperature and pulse rate, I recommend exploring my book "Test Your Thyroid Function."

Chapter 4: Pro-Metabolic Diet

The "Ray Peat Diet"

A significant portion of Dr. Ray Peat's research revolves around the interactions between nutrition, hormones, and health. His research underscores the crucial role of proper nutrition in maintaining optimal thyroid function and hormonal health.

Although Dr. Peat has not specified an exact diet plan, his nutritional recommendations have evolved over the years, and today, those who follow his dietary principles refer to it as the "Ray Peat diet".

Upon my initial interaction with Dr. Ray Peat, he recommended avoiding certain foods such as polyunsaturated fats, beans, lentils, nuts, seeds, soy products, and raw vegetables from the cabbage (cruciferous) family, due to their potential to substantially inhibit thyroid function (Peat, 2001a, p. 75; Peat, 2001d, p. 17).

In the time since, I've gained knowledge about a multitude of foods, dietary supplements, and other environmental factors that negatively impact thyroid activity and hormonal health.

The "Ray Peat" diet's primary goal is to enhance the body's health by removing foods that obstruct metabolism, and instead, integrating exclusively thyroid-supportive foods into the diet.

In this chapter, I will highlight the most meaningful dietary changes I implemented when I began adhering to Dr. Ray Peat's nutritional guidance. Instead of delving into complex biochemical explanations, I will provide a broad overview of the core principles of the "Ray Peat diet".

Healthy Fats

One major change I made in my diet involved adjusting the kinds of fats I was eating.

Dr. Ray Peat explained that unsaturated fats, prevalent in liquid cooking oils such as corn, canola, soybean, safflower, sunflower, flaxseed, sesame, and peanut oil, negatively impact thyroid function (Peat, 2001b, p. 154).

According to Peat, unsaturated fats hinder thyroid function at multiple stages, including the production of thyroid hormones in the gland, the transportation of these hormones in the bloodstream, as well as the tissue's response to the active thyroid hormone T3 (Peat, 2001b, p. 178; Peat, 2001d, p. iii).

Dr. Ray Peat suggested that I use saturated fats, like coconut oil and butter, instead of the usual cooking oils (Peat, 2001b, p. 157). Over time, I started feeling better with the shift to saturated fats, and I think this change really helped improve my thyroid function.

High-Quality Protein

Dr. Ray Peat emphasized the importance of consuming high-quality protein for maintaining optimal thyroid health. He pointed out that the liver requires a considerable amount of protein to carry out its vital functions, such as converting the storage hormone T4 to the active thyroid hormone T3 (Peat, 2001a, pp. 73-74; Peat, 2001d, p. 96).

Dr. Peat expressed a preference for animal protein over plant-based protein sources such as beans, lentils, nuts, and soy products. He explained that humans often struggle to digest and extract protein from plant-based sources. Additionally, beans, lentils, nuts, and soy products contain high amounts of unsaturated fats, estrogens, and other compounds that can suppress thyroid function (Peat, 2001d, p. 17; Peat, 2001b, pp. 19-20).

Peat recommended sourcing high-quality protein from animal-based foods like cheese, milk, eggs, shellfish, beef, lamb, low-fat fish, and gelatin. Although meat from ruminant animals is part of Peat's dietary guidelines, he warned that eating too much muscle meat could lead to an unfavorable ratio of anti-thyroid amino acids (Peat, 2001d, p. 81). On the other hand, gelatin provides a more thyroid-friendly amino acid profile. Thus, gelatinous cuts of meat and gelatin powder are components of the "Ray Peat diet" (Peat, 2004, p. 1).

A key feature of the "Ray Peat diet" is the inclusion of shellfish such as shrimp, oysters, clams, mussels, scallops, and lobster. These foods offer high-quality protein and essential trace minerals that support thyroid function (Wilson, 2015, p. 26; Peat, 2001b, pp. 171-172).

Many people wonder if it's possible to follow the "Ray Peat diet" as a vegan or vegetarian. Some plant-based protein sources, like well-cooked white button mushrooms and potatoes, can provide quality protein similar to animal sources (Peat, 2001d, p. 99). Thus, following Dr. Ray Peat's diet protocol as a vegan is doable but challenging. It may be easier as a vegetarian since it allows for the inclusion of protein from milk, cheese, and eggs.

By basing one's diet on large amounts of milk and cheese, there are added benefits of high calcium intake, which, according to Dr. Ray Peat, is vital for good health (Peat, 2001d, p. 81).

After ensuring I consumed sufficient high-quality protein in my daily diet, I noticed immediate health benefits. However, it's important to mention that it's essential to eat protein alongside healthy carbohydrates, which will be discussed in more detail later in this chapter.

Important Carbohydrates

Despite the common advice from dietitians and doctors to limit sugar intake, leading many people to avoid not only sugars but also fruits, Dr. Ray Peat provided a different perspective.

Peat encouraged the consumption of carbohydrates from well-cooked vegetables like potatoes and advocated for a generous intake of orange juice and low-starch, sweet fruits such as melons, grapes, and tropical fruits (Peat, 2001d, p. 95; Peat, 2001d, p. iv). Milk and cheese, being rich in milk sugar, also make excellent carbohydrate sources. Surprisingly, even honey and white sugar have their place in the "Ray Peat diet". It's worth noting that fruits and honey, unlike white sugar, also supply essential minerals (Peat, 2001b, p. 189).

Before discovering Peat's nutritional principles, I, too, was following a low-sugar diet. However, Peat enlightened me to the concept that sugars aren't our enemy. He underscored that our liver needs sugar, just as it requires protein, to function optimally (Peat, 2001a, pp. 73-74). Glucose is crucial for the liver's conversion of T4 into the active thyroid hormone T3, and the metabolic rate can significantly decrease during fasting periods. Experimental studies suggest that adding 200 to 300 calories of carbohydrates to our diet doesn't typically lead to fat storage (Peat, 2001a, p. 73).

If an individual exhibits elevated T4 levels yet continues to experience symptoms of hypothyroidism, it might be because T4 isn't being converted to T3 (Peat, 2001a, p. 74). This issue could potentially be addressed through dietary changes. Incorporating a piece of fruit, or a glass of orange juice or milk between meals can stimulate the liver to produce the T3 hormone (Peat, 2001a, p. 74).

When I first encountered Dr. Ray Peat, I was dealing with severe hypoglycemia (low blood sugar), a condition that made it exceedingly challenging for me to consume sugary foods and starches as they would severely disrupt my blood sugar levels, triggering hypoglycemic episodes. Initially, I couldn't include white sugar in my diet, but incorporating sweet fruits and orange juice significantly improved my low blood sugar condition. This change was transformative for me. Additionally, under Dr. Ray Peat's guidance, I learned how to effectively combine foods, which further helped alleviate my low blood sugar problem over time.

Balanced Meals

Dr. Ray Peat explained that consuming considerable amounts of protein (such as from eggs and meat) or starches (like bread, pasta, and rice) independently may cause symptoms of low blood sugar, including dizziness, headaches, and fatigue (Peat, 2001d, p. iv; Peat, 2001d, p. 95).

Peat taught me that balanced meals featuring healthy carbohydrates, quality protein, and saturated fats can steady blood sugar levels, stabilize stress hormones, and increase thyroid function (Peat, 2001b, p. 189). Balanced meals are not only important for people with low blood sugar issues, but the general recommendation of Dr. Ray Peat (Peat, 2001d, p. 95).

Ingesting small snacks between meals, such as sweet fruits, orange juice, milk, or cheese, can aid in maintaining steady blood sugar levels and a consistent metabolic rate throughout the day (Peat, 2001d, p. iv). Foods like cheese and milk, which are sources of both fat, sugar, and protein, are balanced meals in themselves and can be consumed individually. Sweet fruits and orange juice also serve as excellent choices for standalone snacks (Peat, 2001d, p. iv; Peat, 2001b, p. 189).

Dr. Ray Peat's Carrot Salad

Dr. Ray Peat recommended a cautious approach toward consuming raw vegetables like salads. He reasoned that our human digestive system finds it challenging to extract nutrients from raw vegetables due to our inability to effectively break down their fibers. Moreover, the indigestible fibers in many raw vegetables may foster the growth of detrimental bacteria in the intestines (Ray Peat Clips, 2016).

Raw carrots are an exception to the general caution against consuming raw vegetables. Peat advocated for the consumption of raw carrots, attributing this to the antimicrobial properties of their fibers (Peat, 2001b, p. 189). His dietary guidelines notably include a "carrot salad," which consists of raw grated carrots eaten with a dressing of olive or coconut oil, vinegar, and salt (Peat, 2001a, p. 105).

According to Peat, raw carrots, particularly in the form of his carrot salad, can aid in intestinal cleansing. The fibers in carrots promote bowel movements, reduce fungal and bacterial overgrowth, minimize estrogen reabsorption, and limit the absorption of bacterial toxins (Peat, 2001b, pp. 40-41).

Consuming Peat's carrot salad daily can potentially improve a person's hormonal balance (Peat, 2001b, p.93). Several individuals have reported improvements in symptoms of PMS, allergies, and headaches with daily consumption of raw carrots (Peat, 2001b, p. 189).

A Note on the "Ray Peat Diet"

At its core, the Ray Peat diet involves consuming healthy saturated fats, such as coconut oil and butter.

Protein sources should come primarily from dairy products, eggs, shellfish, low-fat fish, collagen-rich meats from ruminant animals, and gelatin powder.

Carbohydrates should primarily come from a variety of sweet fruits, orange juice, and thoroughly cooked vegetables, with a particular emphasis on potatoes.
It is vital to maintain a balance of fats, proteins, and carbohydrates in each meal, and it is recommended to have small snacks of fruit, orange juice, milk, or cheese between main meals. Additionally, the daily consumption of a raw carrot or Dr. Ray Peat's carrot salad is helpful (Peat, 2001b, pp. 188-199).

The "Ray Peat diet" is often sought out by individuals looking to enhance their thyroid function and hormonal balance. However, this diet is also beneficial for anyone striving for optimal health (Howley, 2023). It ensures the body receives all essential nutrients while avoiding energy-suppressing compounds, such as unsaturated fats (Howley, 2023; Peat, 2001b, pp. 175-183).

Upon studying Dr. Ray Peat's dietary principles, I came to appreciate his unique approach. The diet includes a variety of enjoyable foods, eliminating any sense of deprivation. Instead of enforcing a strict regimen, it provides a comprehensive understanding of dietary principles that support metabolism.

In my exploration of Dr. Ray Peat's research, I gained a clear understanding of the connection between nutrition and metabolism. I discovered that adopting his pro-metabolic dietary principles is a crucial first step in improving thyroid function. If you're undergoing thyroid replacement therapy, selecting the right diet is particularly important, as an unsuitable diet can hinder the effectiveness of the medication. Conversely, following the "Ray Peat diet" works synergistically with thyroid therapy to alleviate symptoms of low thyroid function and promote the body's healing process.

It's important to emphasize that Dr. Ray Peat's nutritional recommendations are rooted in a deep understanding of the body's biochemical processes. This makes it easier to stick with the diet long-term, as you comprehend the reasons behind each recommendation.

In my third book, "How To Boost Metabolism With Food," you can gain a deeper understanding of Dr.

Ray Peat's dietary research, along with precise recommendations on which foods to avoid and which to include for a pro-metabolic lifestyle.

Chapter 5: Thyroid Replacement Therapy

Best Thyroid Medication

To overcome hypothyroidism, using the appropriate type of thyroid medication and consuming it correctly has been critical for me.

Prior to connecting with Dr. Ray Peat, I had been on different types of prescription thyroid medications.

However, I faced several challenges, and my symptoms persisted, due to my inadequate understanding of how to effectively utilize the medication. My perspective changed significantly upon contacting Dr. Ray Peat.

Following Peat's guidance, I comprehended that the most effective thyroid medication is a combination of T4 and T3 hormones, consumed in a ratio of approximately 3:1, mirroring the secretion pattern of the human thyroid gland (Peat, 2001a, p.73). This can be achieved via synthetic hormones or natural desiccated thyroid (NDT), which is an animal thyroid extract (Peat, 2000, pp.5-6). I have successfully used both natural desiccated thyroid and synthetic thyroid hormones.

In this chapter, I will outline crucial aspects of thyroid medication, based on what Dr. Ray Peat shared with me.

Problems with T4 Therapy

The standard treatment for individuals diagnosed with hypothyroidism typically involves administering a synthetic form of T4, known as levothyroxine. Levothyroxine is available under several brand names such as Synthroid, Levoxyl, Unithroid, and Tirosint in the United States, and Euthyrox and Eltroxin in Europe (Jonklaas et al., 2014 pp. 1670-1751).

In numerous articles and interviews, Dr. Ray Peat has emphasized the potential complications arising from a treatment regimen relying solely on T4 (Peat, 2001a, pp.73-74).

T4 must be converted into T3, a process primarily occurring in the liver (Peat, 2001a, pp.73-74). However, as previously explained, this conversion can be compromised in certain individuals due to factors such as impaired liver function, low blood sugar, stress, the wrong diet etc. (Peat, 2008, pp.3-5; Wilson, 2015, pp.24-28).

Consequently, individuals with insufficient conversion from T4 to T3 may continue to exhibit symptoms of hypothyroidism despite being on levothyroxine (Wilson, 2015, pp.24-28).

Dr. Ray Peat elaborated on how this predicament escalates when these individuals increase their dosage of levothyroxine. If T4 is not converted into T3, it accumulates in tissues, and at a certain point, it starts exerting anti-thyroid effects (Peat, 2000, p.5). Therefore, increasing the dosage of levothyroxine can sometimes intensify the symptoms of hypothyroidism (Wilson, 2015, p.27; Peat, 2000, p.5).

Due to the problems with T4 treatment, Dr. Ray Peat supported the use of combination therapy involving both T4 and T3.

T4 + T3 Combination Therapy

There are other proponents of T3 treatment for individuals with low thyroid levels, apart from Dr. Peat. Dr. Denis Wilson, an American physician, is one such advocate who stresses the importance of T3 in the management of hypothyroidism (Wilson, 2015, pp. 24-28).

Dr. Ray Peat advocated for balanced thyroid therapy with both T4 and T3, consumed in a ratio of approximately 3:1, mirroring the secretion pattern of the human thyroid gland (Peat, 2001a, p.73; Peat, 2001a, p.105).

In the rest of this chapter, I will delve deeper into Dr. Ray Peat's guidelines regarding thyroid replacement therapy.

Natural versus Synthetic

Natural Desiccated Thyroid (NDT), or thyroid extract, is a product derived from the dried and powdered thyroid gland of an animal, usually a pig (porcine thyroid) or a cow (bovine thyroid) (Peat, 2000, p. 5).

Before the advent of synthetic hormones, thyroid extracts were the initial form of thyroid replacement therapy and remain in use today for treating hypothyroidism (Peat, 2000, pp. 5-7).

A high-quality thyroid extract releases a T4 to T3 ratio of approximately 3:1 upon digestion, closely mimicking the secretion pattern of the human thyroid gland (Peat, 2000, p. 5; Peat, 2001a, p. 73).

Thyroid extracts are available as prescription drugs, such as Armour thyroid, and in some countries also as over-the-counter supplements (Peat, 2001d, p. 18).

With technological advancements, synthetic thyroid hormones have been synthesized, offering combination pills containing both T4 (levothyroxine) and T3 (liothyronine). Furthermore, a T3 medication can be combined with a T4 medication to achieve the preferred T4 to T3 ratio (Peat, 2000, pp. 5-6).

Synthetic hormones are quantified in micrograms (mcg), whereas natural desiccated thyroid is measured in milligrams (mg) or grains, with one grain equating to 60 mg of thyroid extract (Peat, 2000, p. 5-6).

Historically, the conventional adult dosage of natural desiccated thyroid was around two grains (120mg) per day (Barnes & Galton, 1976, p. 282-286).
Synthetic combination thyroid pills often employ a four-to-one T4 to T3 ratio, with a blend of 100 mcg of T4 and 25 mcg of T3, said to equate to about two grains of natural desiccated thyroid (Peat, 2000, p. 5).

Although this ratio is sufficient for many, some individuals require a higher proportion of T3 for optimal results. T3 proves especially beneficial in early treatment stages, aiding the liver's functionality (Peat, 2000, p. 6).

Starting thyroid medication can be a bit tricky, especially if you've been dealing with low thyroid function for a long time.

Peat made it clear to me that it's best to slowly increase to your final dosage over time. He pointed out that if you start with what you think will be your final dose right away, you might end up feeling some negative side effects (Peat, 2000, p. 6).

Considering that T4 gradually builds up in your tissues, the full effect of a given thyroid dosage isn't seen until about two weeks, when the T4 levels reach a steady state (Peat, 2000, p. 6). It may take several months for the body to adapt to a higher metabolic rate, and consequently, achieving the optimal dosage of thyroid replacement therapy can be a lengthy process (Peat, 2000, p. 6).

T3 is a potent hormone that works immediately, it has a short half-life, which means it doesn't build up in the body like T4 does (Peat, 2000, p. 6). A typical, healthy human body produces around four mcg of T3 per hour, which totals to approximately 100 mcg daily (Taper, 2012). Taking an overly large dose of T3 at once is not in line with the body's natural physiological function, and could lead to negative side effects. Furthermore, the body may deactivate some of the excessive T3 to protect itself (Peat, 2001a, p. 74).

Any thyroid medication, whether natural or synthetic, containing T3 should therefore be distributed into several doses to be consumed across the day (Peat, 2000, pp. 5-6; Ray Peat Clips, 2021).

Peat also recommended administering your thyroid product with food to further delay the absorption of T3 and simulate the body's steady production of T3.

This advice deviates from the common suggestion of taking thyroid medication on an empty stomach (Ray Peat Clips, 2021).

Dr. Ray Peat taught me that it's crucial to carefully monitor your body's response to thyroid replacement therapy, regardless of whether it is natural or synthetic. This is due to potential potency issues that could arise from manufacturing inconsistencies. If a specific form of thyroid replacement therapy proved to be ineffective, Dr. Ray Peat suggested exploring alternatives, such as transitioning from a natural to a synthetic form or trying a different brand.

By leveraging the insights, I acquired from Dr. Ray Peat, I was able to use my thyroid medications effectively and incrementally increase my metabolic rate.

It's critical to recognize that improper use of thyroid replacement therapy can lead to various complications. While I do not prescribe medication, I regularly assist individuals who are on thyroid medication through my counseling services. My goal is to offer information and insights, aiding in the effective management of their thyroid replacement therapy.

Chapter 6: Hormonal Support

Youth Associated Hormones

Upon first meeting Dr. Ray Peat, I quickly realized that he not only possessed extensive knowledge about thyroid function but also had a deep understanding of hormones in general.

According to Dr. Peat's teachings, a healthy human body requires both optimal thyroid function and sufficient levels of the steroid hormones: Pregnenolone, progesterone, and dehydroepiandrosterone (DHEA) (Peat, 2001a, pp. 68-69). These natural hormones possess anti-aging and anti-stress properties and are referred to as youth-associated hormones since they are abundant during youth (Peat, 2001b, pp. 71-75).

The body produces the youth-associated hormones by initially converting cholesterol into pregnenolone. Enzymes can then convert pregnenolone into either progesterone or DHEA (Peat, 2001a, pp. 68-69). Optimal production of pregnenolone from cholesterol relies on the presence of the active thyroid hormone (T3) and the retinol form of vitamin A (Peat, 2001b, p. 69). Consequently, inadequate thyroid function and the wrong diet can result in diminished levels of youth-associated hormones (Peat, 2001a, pp. 68-69).

Dr. Peat enlightened me about the potential benefits of supplementing with pregnenolone and progesterone when there may be a deficiency of these hormones, such as during periods of stress, illness, hypothyroidism, inflammation, PMS, menopause, and aging (Peat, 2001b, pp. 71-75).

Supplementing with progesterone and pregnenolone can help optimize thyroid function and alleviate stress by rebalancing excessive levels of estrogen and cortisol (Peat, 2001b, pp. 67-69).
During my recovery from hypothyroidism and hormonal imbalances, I incorporated both of these natural hormones into my supplementation regimen.

Pregnenolone played a particularly vital role at the beginning of my recovery as it helped me manage the stress of increasing my metabolic rate and enabled me to augment my thyroid medication without experiencing adverse side effects.

In the rest of this chapter, I will outline important aspects of progesterone and pregnenolone supplementation as taught to me by Dr. Ray Peat.

Benefits of Progesterone

Dr. Ray Peat extensively researched the hormone progesterone and has authored several books and published numerous articles on the topic.

Peat's findings indicate that progesterone is the most protective hormone naturally produced by the human body (Peat, 2001b, pp. 71-72). Progesterone functions as a direct antagonist to estrogen, meaning it exerts opposite effects to estrogen (Peat, 2001c, pp. 4-8). His research highlights the many benefits of progesterone for human health, including its ability to reduce stress and inflammation, alleviate PMS symptoms, support healthy pregnancies, enhance fertility, improve sleep, alleviate menopause symptoms, and boost thyroid and immune function, among others (Peat, 2001c, pp. 60-61).

Peat suggested the use of a supplement containing 10% progesterone dissolved in vitamin E. In this particular form, progesterone is roughly 20 times more potent compared to other preparations, highlighting the significance of utilizing it in suitable physiological quantities (Peat, 2001a, p. 70).

When taken orally, this 10% progesterone supplement is efficiently absorbed and rapidly distributed throughout the body's tissues (Peat,

2001b, p. 72). It's important to note that high dosages of progesterone without estrogen opposition have a sedative effect, emphasizing the need to determine the minimum effective dosage (Peat, 2001a, p. 70; Peat, 2001c, p. 39).

While progesterone is naturally produced by men and progesterone supplementation can provide benefits in some cases, it is not classified as a male hormone (Peat, 2001b, p. 72). Women should use progesterone cyclically, typically for two weeks per month, starting just after ovulation and continuing until menstruation. Even for women who do not menstruate, cycling progesterone is recommended, especially when higher dosages are used (Peat, 2001c, p. 39).

Benefits of Pregnenolone

Before meeting Dr. Ray Peat, I had never been introduced to the concept of pregnenolone supplementation. However, I swiftly discovered the immense value of this supplement.

According to Peat, pregnenolone is abundantly present in young individuals of both sexes and serves as a vital defense against hormonal imbalances (Peat, 2001b, p. 73). Similar to progesterone, it safeguards against the detrimental effects of excessive estrogen and cortisone (Peat, 2001b, p. 73). Pregnenolone also tends to enhance the functioning of the thyroid and other glands, exerting a "normalizing" influence that accounts for its broad spectrum of beneficial effects (Peat, 2001b, p. 74).

Notably, pregnenolone shields brain cells from fatigue-induced injury and possesses a calming effect on emotions. It improves skin circulation, joint mobility, tissue elasticity, eyesight, and more (Peat, 2001b, p. 73). Moreover, in cases where an individual is experiencing elevated cortisone levels due to stress, adequate pregnenolone intake helps restore cortisone to normal levels (Peat, 2001b, p. 73).

Pregnenolone is suitable for both men and women, and its powdered form is reasonably well-absorbed when taken orally (Peat, 2001b, p. 73). It can be used on an as-needed basis or taken daily, depending on personal preference. Peat discovered that if the pregnenolone source is pure and of high quality, there are no adverse side effects from pregnenolone, even when taken in significantly large dosages (Peat, 2001b, p. 113).

A Note on Hormonal Support

Gaining a comprehensive understanding of progesterone and pregnenolone supplements is crucial prior to their utilization. It is important to be knowledgeable about recommended dosages, and considerations for specific health conditions.

It is essential to note that while progesterone and pregnenolone are available as over-the-counter supplements in the United States, they may be classified as medications in other countries. Therefore, it is crucial to thoroughly educate yourself about the laws and guidelines of your country regarding these natural hormones before considering their utilization.

If obtaining progesterone and pregnenolone is not feasible or if you prefer to abstain from supplementing with these substances, there are alternative methods to enhance the body's natural production of pregnenolone and progesterone. This can be achieved by optimizing thyroid function, maintaining adequate cholesterol levels, ensuring sufficient vitamin A intake from your diet or through supplementation, and receiving ample exposure to appropriate types of light.

Chapter 7: Nutritional Supplements

Risk and Benefits of Supplements

When I initially spoke with Dr. Ray Peat, I was taking various nutritional supplements. However, he warned me about the potential risks associated with some of these supplements.

Firstly, I learned that many pills and capsules contain additives and fillers that can be absorbed by the body, leading to negative health effects (Peat, 2001d, pp. 77-80).

Additionally, I came to understand that I should discontinue supplementing with fish oils, iron, iodine, carotene, flax seeds, seed oils, and also stop my mega-dosing of the amino acids tryptophan and glutamic acid. Dr. Peat explained that these supplements have the potential to trigger inflammation, suppress the immune system, disrupt hormonal balance, and have adverse effects on the thyroid.

Dr. Peat recommended obtaining vitamins and minerals from nutrient-rich foods rather than heavily relying on supplements. His dietary principles emphasize the importance of consuming foods such as orange juice, liver, eggs, milk, cheese, shellfish, and cooked greens. These foods not only support metabolism but also provide an abundance of essential vitamins and minerals.

While some supplements can be detrimental, others can be beneficial. Dr. Ray Peat emphasized the therapeutic benefits of specific nutritional supplements, including vitamin A, vitamin E, vitamin D, vitamin K, niacinamide (vitamin B3), thiamine (vitamin B1), calcium carbonate, and aspirin. Additionally, individual needs may require supplementation with other essential vitamins and minerals (Peat, 2001d, pp. 92-93).

During his research, Dr. Ray Peat dedicated significant effort to exploring the health benefits of different compounds. In his newsletters and interviews, he often emphasized the advantageous properties of various substances and superfoods, highlighting their anti-aging, anti-inflammatory, and energy-supporting effects. Personally, I have successfully incorporated several of these into my own health routine and now educate my clients about the benefits they offer.

Based on my experience as a nutritional and metabolic counselor, I have observed that many individuals consume a significant number of daily supplements, some of which can have detrimental effects on their health.

It is crucial to acknowledge that navigating the supplement market can be challenging due to the prevalence of products with misleading claims. As discussed in this chapter, numerous commonly promoted supplements can do more harm than good.

In my work with clients, I take great care to thoroughly assess their supplement regimen and educate them about the potential risks associated with commonly used supplements. When appropriate, I assist clients in identifying the purest and most effective products available on the market.

Chapter 8: Light Therapy

Benedicte Mai Lerche MSc PhD

Light, Hormones, and Health

Niels Ryberg Finsen and John Harvey Kellogg were both pioneers in the field of light therapy and recognized the therapeutic benefits of sunlight (Loignon, 2022, p. 103-128).

Niels Ryberg Finsen (1860-1904) was a Danish physician and scientist who made significant contributions to the field of phototherapy, meaning the use of light to treat disease. He founded the Finsen Institute for Phototherapy in Copenhagen in 1896, and he was awarded the Nobel Prize in Medicine in 1903 for his work (Nobel Media AB, 2021).

John Harvey Kellogg (1852-1943) was an American physician, and health reformer who advocated for the use of natural remedies and lifestyle changes to promote good health (Loignon, 2022, p. 103). Kellogg is credited with inventing the breakfast cereal known as "Corn Flakes". He also used light therapy in his work (Loignon, 2022, p. 103).

While Finsen's work focused on the use of certain wavelengths of light to treat specific medical conditions, Kellogg believed that exposure to sunlight and the use of light therapy could have a more general therapeutic effect on the body (Loignon, 2022, p. 123).

Both Finsen and Kellogg developed specialized lamps and devices to deliver light therapy, and their work paved the way for further research and development within this field (Loignon, 2022, pp. 103-128).

Light therapy has had a long tradition in medicine. Although it has fallen somewhat out of favor over the past decades, there has been a renewed interest in recent times (Liebert & Kiat, 2021, p. 389).

Dr. Ray Peat was also very interested in the benefits of sunlight and light therapy. He explained that prolonged darkness can be very stressful for the body, as it increases the production of the stress hormone cortisol, which in turn can promote degenerative processes in the body (Peat, 2001a, pp. 76-81).

Peat also emphasized that people tend to be healthier in the summer (Peat, 2001b, pp. 144-150). He explained that it is the red and orange wavelengths of sunlight which is so beneficial (Peat, 2001b, p. 149). These rays can penetrate deep into the body's tissues, where they help promote energy production, and tends to normalize (or maximize) the production of beneficial hormones, including progesterone and the thyroid hormones (Peat, 2001a, p. 18; Peat, 2001c, p. 37).

Peat advocated for getting plenty of sunlight, although he stressed that you should avoid sunburn (Peat, 2001b, pp. 144-150). In regions with limited sunlight, he suggested utilizing light therapy lamps to access the beneficial orange and red wavelengths of light (Peat, 2001b, pp. 144-150).

Residing in Denmark, where winters tend to be lengthy, I have opted to utilize specific light therapy lamps that offer me the red and orange wavelengths of light. Although it is crucial to emphasize that light therapy and sunlight cannot cure severe hypothyroidism, I have observed positive effects on my health.

Chapter 9: Full Recovery

Unlocking Optimal Health

After adopting Dr. Ray Peat's health methodology, I experienced significant health improvements within a few months. Symptoms such as fatigue, headaches, muscle pain, low blood sugar, and digestive issues were drastically reduced. My cholesterol levels normalized, and my polycystic ovarian syndrome vanished, resulting in the return of my menstrual cycle.

Within about four months, I felt well enough to resume my studies in Biochemistry at the University of Copenhagen. My studies deepened my understanding of the scientific basis behind Dr. Ray Peat's health recommendations, and by consistently following his advice, I was able to achieve further progress and eventually became symptom-free.

It is important to note that Dr. Ray Peat's health method is not a quick fix but a long-term approach to maintaining good health throughout one's life. Peat believed that disease is created when there is a gap between the body's energy resources and the demands of the environment. He explained that a pro-metabolic diet and lifestyle have to be consciously chosen to sustain health.

Since discovering Dr. Ray Peat's research, I have followed his principles and feel healthier than ever. Childhood issues such as allergies and eczema have resolved, and I believe that my body has reached its maximum energy potential.

Today I share Dr. Ray Peat's health principles with others who suffer from low thyroid function and hormonal imbalances, with the goal of making his theories accessible to those without a scientific background.

Afterword

As you reach the end of this book, I hope you have found inspiration and guidance on your journey toward healing hypothyroidism. Understanding the complexities of low thyroid function and hormonal imbalances is a crucial first step in reclaiming your well-being.

Consider this book the beginning of your journey into thyroid health and Dr. Ray Peat's remarkable research. While it serves as an introduction to his groundbreaking work, much more awaits discovery. My 'Healing Metabolism' book series aims to expand on the health principles introduced here, with each subsequent book exploring a specific subject in greater depth.

If you are seeking additional information, resources, and support, I invite you to visit my website, biochemnordic.com. There, you will find a wealth of supplementary content and tools to deepen your understanding and assist you in implementing the principles discussed in this book.

It is important to emphasize that this book has presented my own experience in overcoming hypothyroidism and hormonal imbalances and that your recovery process might differ from mine.

Remember, metabolic and hormonal regeneration is a process that demands dedication, patience, and a commitment to self-care.

Embrace the knowledge you have gained through this book and take the necessary steps to incorporate positive changes into your life.

I sincerely thank you for accompanying me on this transformative path. May your future be filled with vibrant health, boundless energy, and the joy of living life to its fullest.

Warmest regards,
Benedicte Mai Lerche

About the Author

Benedicte Mai Lerche earned an MSc in Biochemistry from the University of Copenhagen and a Ph.D. in Chemical and Biochemical Engineering from the Technical University of Denmark.

Benedicte is deeply committed to assisting individuals in overcoming challenges associated with low thyroid function and hormonal imbalances.

Through her website, biochemnordic.com, she offers a vast array of e-learning materials and personalized video counseling, designed to assist individuals globally on their health journey.

Another contribution to her extensive collection of resources is the "Healing Metabolism" book series. This particular book represents the first volume in this significant series.

With a primary focus on supporting optimal thyroid function and boosting cellular energy production, Benedicte shares invaluable knowledge on dietary principles, supplement recommendations, and lifestyle factors that promote efficient metabolism and hormone balance, while also offering anti-aging, anti-stress, and anti-inflammatory benefits.

Driven by the profound impact of Dr. Ray Peat's extensive research, Benedicte has personally witnessed the transformative power of his insights in addressing her own thyroid and hormonal struggles. This experience has fueled her dedication to impart Dr. Peat's invaluable knowledge to others who are encountering similar issues.

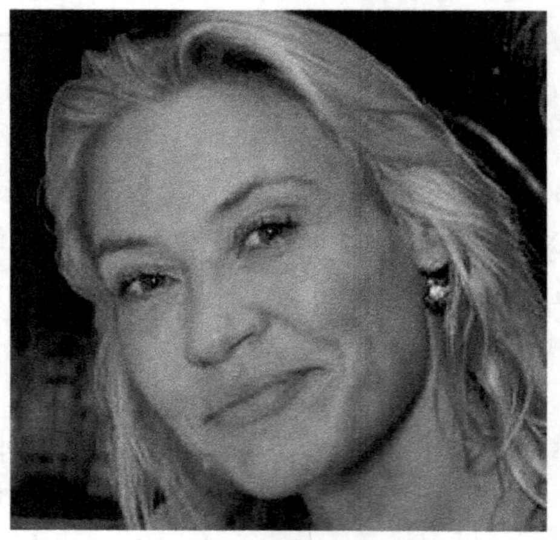

Benedicte Mai Lerche MSc PhD

Your Review Matters

If you found this book valuable, I would be immensely grateful if you could take a moment to leave a review on the platform where you purchased the book or on Goodreads.

Your feedback will help other potential readers facing similar health challenges to discover and benefit from my work.

Just a few thoughtful lines from you can make a significant impact.

Thank you sincerely for your support!

Benedicte Mai Lerche

References

Barnes, B., & Galton, L. (1976). *Hypothyroidism The Unsuspected Illness.* HarperCollins.

Faix, J. D. (2013, May 1). *Thyroid-Stimulating Hormone | AACC.org.* From American Association for Clinical Chemistry: https://www.aacc.org/cln/articles/2013/may/tsh-harmonization

Howley, E. K. (2023, March). *What Is the Ray Peat Diet?* From U.S. News & World Report: https://health.usnews.com/wellness/food/article/what-is-the-ray-peat-diet

Jonklaas, J., Bianco, A. C., Bauer, A. J., Burman, K. D., Cappola, A. R., Celi, F. S., . . . Sawka, A. M. (2014). Guidelines for the treatment of hypothyroidism: Prepared by the American thyroid association task force on thyroid hormone replacement. *Thyroid, 24*(12), 1670–1751.

Liebert, A., & Kiat, H. (2021). The history of light therapy in hospital physiotherapy and medicine with emphasis on Australia: Evolution into novel areas of practice. *Physiotherapy Theory and Practice, 37*(3), 389-400.

Loignon, A. E. (2022). Bringing Light to the World: John Harvey Kellogg and Transatlantic Light

Therapy. *Journal of Transatlantic Studies*, 20, 103–128.

Nobel Media AB. (2021). Niels Ryberg Finsen - Biographical. NobelPrize.org. From https://www.nobelprize.org/prizes/medicine/1903/finsen/biographical/

Peat, R. (2000, May). Thyroid: Therapies, Confusion, and Fraud. *Ray Peat's Newsletter*, 1-7.

Peat, R. (2001a). *Generative Energy: Restoring the* Wholeness of Life. Raymond Peat PH.D.

Peat, R. (2001b). From PMS to Menopause: Female Hormones in Context. Raymond Peat PH.D.

Peat, R. (2001c). Progesterone in Orthomolecular Medicine. Raymond Peat PH.D.

Peat, R. (2001d). Nutrition for Women: 100 Short Articles. Raymond Peat PH.D.

Peat, R. (2004, January). Gelatin, stress, longevity. *Ray Peat's newsletter*, 1-8.

Peat, R. (2008, January). TSH, temperature, pulse rate, and other indicators in hypothyroidism. *Ray Peat's Newsletter*, 2-6.

Ray Peat Clips. (2016, October 16). Ray Peat on salads, raw vegetables. From https://www.youtube.com/watch?v=Ni0_iTowDoE

Ray Peat Clips. (2021, September 2). Ray Peat on Dosing T3. From YouTube: https://www.youtube.com/watch?v=P9A8ap4TU2c

Society of Endocrinology. (2020, January). Thyroid Gland. United Kingdom. From You and Your Hormones: https://www.yourhormones.info/glands/thyroid-gland/

Taper, G. (2012, March 25). *Ray Peat, PhD on Thyroid, Temperature, Pulse, and TSH – Functional Performance Systems (FPS).* Retrieved April 12, 2023 from Functional Performance Systems: https://www.functionalps.com/blog/2012/03/25/ray-peat-phd-on-thyroid-temperature-pulse-and-tsh/

Vander, A. J., Sherman, J. H., & Luciano, D. S. (2001). *Human Physiology: The Mechanisms of Body Function.* McGraw-Hill.

Wiersinga, W. M., Duntas, L., Fadeyev, V., Nygaard, B., & Vanderpump, M. P. (2012). 2012 ETA guidelines: The use of L-T4+ L-T3 in the treatment of hypothyroidism. *European thyroid journal, 1*(2), 55-71.

Wilson, D. (2015, June). Low Body Temperature as an Indicator for Poor Expression of Thyroid Hormone. (C. Gustafson, Ed.) *Integrative Medicine, 14*(3), 24–28.

Visit
BiochemNordic.com